Anemia among women of reproductive age: A hidden misery

Maternal anemia: A preventable cause of mortality in developing world

Sumera Aziz Ali
Savera Aziz Ali
Nadir Suhail

ELIVA PRESS

ELIVA PRESS

Sumera Aziz

Savera Aziz Ali

Nadir Suhail

Anemia is one of the major public health issues among women of reproductive age as it leads to high maternal and infant morbidity, and mortality mainly in low-middle income countries. Around 528.7 million (29.4%) women of reproductive age are anemic, of which 20.2 million women are severely anemic. South-East Asia demonstrates a high burden of anemia among women (41.9%), followed by African and Eastern Mediterranean regions with a prevalence of 41.9% and 37.8%, respectively. Anemia can lead to multiple adverse consequences by impairing oxygen delivery to the fetus resulting in intrauterine growth retardation, stillbirths, preterm births, low birth weight and neonatal deaths.

Published: Eliva Press SRL
Address: MD-2060, bd.Cuza-Voda, 1/4, of. 21 Chişinău, Republica Moldova
Email: info@elivapress.com
Website: www.elivapress.com

ISBN: 978-1-952751-30-1

Contents

Chapter 1: Historical perspective of iron deficiency anemia

Overview of Chlorosis/Hypochromic Anemia

Chlorosis was a prevalent disease during the eighteenth and ninetieth centuries and is now believed to be iron deficiency anemia (Starobinski, 1981). The name chlorosis is derived from the Greek word *chloros*, meaning green (Guggenheim, 1995). During the seventeenth century (1615), one of the Professors of Medicine at Montpellier, Dr. Jean Varandal, suggested this name due to a greenish shade discerned on his patients' skin (Mettler, 1947). Thus, a popular English term, "green sickness," became famous for chlorosis during the seventeenth and eighteenth centuries. Hypochromic or iron deficiency anemia was historically known as chlorosis or green sickness not only because of the distinct green skin shade, but also due to other symptoms similar to anemia (Loudon, 1980). For instance, patients suffering from chlorosis presented with symptoms such as lack of energy, shortness of breath, indigestion, loss of appetite, and constipation (Loudon, 1980).

Chlorosis was considered as a curse of adolescent and young females until approximately the second to the third decade of the twentieth century (Patek & Heath, 1936). Physicians anticipated to see chlorosis in adolescent girls during the process of sexual maturation and these young girls learned about this disease from family members, friends, media, and their clinicians (Brumberg, 1982). There are numerous references to this disease in literature and art from the sixteenth to the nineteenth centuries. In addition, French, German and English physicians have published several clinical accounts of chlorosis in the literature.

Chlorosis was regarded as anemia of adolescent girls without definite etiology, which commonly occurred in the pauper inhabitants' living under poor hygienic conditions but not completely sparing their counterparts (Loudon, 1984). Sometimes, chlorosis was not even considered a separate disease;rather, it was applied as a label to different degenerative or debilitating diseases such as phthisis (Loudon, 1980). But the clinical accounts and descriptions were consistent having enough diagnostic features to distinguish chlorosis from other common enervating disorders at least up to mid of nineteenth century (Starobinski, 1981). Different physicians provided multiple explanations for the cause of chlorosis but there was no general consensus on the etiology of the disease until the development of hematology and the usage of iron therapy (Stockman, 1895). Hence, in this paper I will analyze how the role of iron therapy in adequate doses and development of hematology helped to re-conceptualize the disease chlorosis to hypochromic anemia among young women.

History of Chlorosis

Dr. Johannes. Lange, a well-known German physician (1485-1566), was the first to describe a malady that may be recognized as hypochromic anemia during the mid of the sixteenth century (1554) (Haden, 1938). Dr. Lange gave a description of a girl as "weak and her face which in the last years was distinguished by rosiness of cheeks and redness of lips, is somehow as if exsanguinated, sadly paled, the heart trembles with every movement of her body and she is seized with dyspnea in dancing and climbing the stairs. Her stomach loathes food, particularly meat" (Major, 1945). After his clinical assessment, Dr. Lange labeled the disease as "morbus virgineus" as it was commonly prevalent among the virgins (Major, 1945). The green color is the best-known sign of chlorosis, but in 1554, Dr. Lange in his original description neither used the term chlorosis, nor did he make any reference to green color in his description (Major, 1945).

Dr. Lange thought that this disease occurred as a result of menstrual blood retention that causes sexual frustration. Therefore, he generally recommended that these young women should get married or live with men and copulate to conceive for better recovery (Major 1945). In more contemporary terms, Dr. Lange considered the condition as psychosomatic due to reduced sexuality, which was thus solved by marriage (Zilborg and Henry 1947). This notion of "morbus virgineus" persisted in some form until the late 19th century (Guggenheim, 1995).

In the seventeenth century, English Physician Dr. Thomas. Sydenham (1624-1689) classified green sickness as a type of hysterical disease (Comrie, 1922; Sydenham, 1718). The word "hystery" is derived from the Greek hysteron meaning uterus (Rand, 1986). The "hystery" was considered a mental disease like mania, epilepsy, melancholy, paranoia, and Dr. Sydenham believed this disease to occur as a consequence of the uterus drifting in the body of a young girl (Zilborg and Henry 1947). He also thought that this hysterical disease was not only limited to adolescent girls, but also found in slim and weak women (Sydenham, 1718). Dr. Sydenham also indicated that this condition is due to weak blood causing a dull color, trembling of the heart, and sometimes confusion of the spirits in severe cases (Sydenham, 1718).

Dr. Sydenham's pronounced contribution in this field was the advocacy of iron as a therapy for chlorosis. He proposed that "the sick must drink some mineral water impregnated with the iron mine" (Sydenham, 1718). Although in the 1600s, it was not yet discovered that iron is an imperative component of blood, but in ancient Greco-Roman medicine, iron was considered as a sign of strength impregnated with force by the god Mars (Christian, 1903). This may have been the rationale for Sydenham's promoting iron as a therapy to revive the devitalized blood and to provide strength to shattered spirits (Christian, 1903). Thus, it was the period in medicine that drug's efficacy was established before discovering its mechanism of action.

Etiology of Chlorosis with Different Explanations

There were numerous diverse views and beliefs regarding the etiology of chlorosis (Siddall, 1982). Initially, this disease was attributed to sexual frustration or love-sickness (King, 2004). This view was generally held until the end of the eighteenth and beginning of the nineteenth century when a combination of environmental, organic, and psychogenic factors was recognized as the reason for chlorosis.

A well-known French pediatrician, Dr. J. Parrot, believed that the disease results from physiological changes occurring in the bodies of adolescent girls at puberty (Guggenheim, 1995). He further explained that maturation of the nervous system causes different symptoms at the time of puberty. This maturation, in turn, stimulates the cardiovascular system to cause palpitations, the respiratory system to cause shortness of breath or dyspnea and the gastrointestinal system to cause epigastric pain, indigestion, and constipation (Guggenheim, 1995). Thus, Dr. J. Parrot considered chlorosis as a neuropathological disease resulting from nervous weakness and the greater sensitivity of females as compared to males (Guggenheim, 1995).

On the other hand, a German physician, Dr. Andrew Clerk believed that chlorotic girls are constipated, which causes retention of noxious substances (ptomaines) created by retained stools, which are absorbed into the blood (Taylor et al., 1896). This in turn break downs red blood cells thus causing alterations in the blood (Taylor et al., 1896). In contrast, Dr. Von Noorden, an

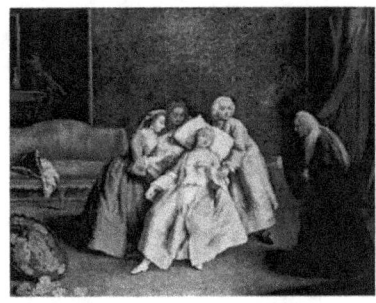

influential German clinician well known for metabolic disease research, had a different belief regarding the etiology of chlorosis. According to Dr. Noorden, chlorosis is caused by the weakness of the blood-forming organs, resulting from a loss of chemical and physiological stimuli originating in the female genitals (Guggenheim, 1995). Based on his explanation for the disease, Dr. Noorden proposed arsenic, iron, and hydrotherapy as different modes of treatment to recuperate the blood-forming organs (Guggenheim, 1995).

On the contrary, Dr. William Osler, a well-known Canadian physician, attributed this disease to the poor environment and lifestyle of the young girls (Osler 1892). He believed that young girls might present with emotional and nervous disturbances, but he did not consider this disease resulting from nervous or psychiatric disorders (Osler 1892). According to Dr. Osler "chlorosis is most common among ill-fed, overworked girls of large towns who are confined all day in close, badly-lighted rooms. Cases are frequent, however, under the most favorable

TABLE I—*Monthly report of diseases[11] admitted under the care of the physicians of the Finsbury Dispensary, St John's Square, Clerkenwell*

List of diseases etc from 20 March to 20 April 1800

Continued fever	16	Nephralgia calculosa	1
Scarlet fever	2	Pleurodyne	3
Measles	1	Hydrops	4
Sore throat	4	Hymorrhis	3
Haemoptysis	4	Hysteria	3
Pulmonary complaints without fever	53	Paralysis	3
Phthisis pulmonalis	12	Apoplexy	1
Dysentery	3	Schrophula	2
Diarrhoea	4	Colica Pictonum	1
Chlorosis and amenorrhoea	29	Hypochondriasis	1
Leucorrhea	7	Insanity	2
Menorrhagia	6	Hooping cough	4
Asthenia	10	Rheumatism	4
Dyspepsia	6	Febricula	4
Enterodynia	2	Febris mesenterica	3
Peritonitis	1	Vermes	8
Constipation	1	Fever infantilis	6
Vertigo	2	Chronic cutaneous diseases	15
Cephalea	5		

5

conditions of life. Lack of proper exercise and fresh air and improper food are important factors" (Osier 1892).

TABLE II—*Number of admissions to dispensaries for amenorrhea and chlorosis, menorrhagia, and all menstrual disorders, expressed as total numbers and as percentages of total medical admissions to the dispensaries*

Date	Dispensary	Admissions for amenorrhea and chlorosis		Admissions for menorrhagia		Admissions for all menstrual disorders		Total medical admissions to the dispensary
		No	%	No	%	No	%	
	London							
1774	General Dispensary[17]	29	1·7	22	1·3	51	3·1	1662
1775-6	The Westminster General[18]	12	0·9	20	1·5	32	2·4	1320
1800	Finsbury Dispensary[19]	128	4·6	74	2·7	202	7·3	2771
1811	Western Dispensary[20]	36	2·8	4	0·3	42	3·3	1283
1801	Public Dispensary[21]	78	2·2	38	1·1	116	3·3	3508
	Provincial							
1804	Liverpool Dispensary[22]	208	2·0	97	0·9	315	2·9	10350
1801	Bath City Dispensary[23]	19	1·5	14	1·1	33	2·6	1222
1808	Plymouth Dispensary[24]	134	3·3	55	1·4	194	4·8	4010
1808	Norwich Dispensary[25]	18	2·9	10	1·6	29	4·7	611
1818	Combined Dublin Dispensaries[26]	285	1·6	165	0·9	450	2·6	17269

TABLE III—*Number of admissions to the outpatient departments of various hospitals for amenorrhea and chlorosis, menorrhagia, and all menstrual disorders, expressed as total numbers and as percentages of all admissions*

Date	Hospital	Admissions for amenorrhea and chlorosis		Admissions for menorrhagia		Admissions for all menstrual disorders		Total admissions
		No	%	No	%	No	%	
1799	Westminster Hospital[27]*	51	4·4	12	1·0	63	5·5	1153
1760	Bristol Infirmary	63	4·2	14	0·9	77	5·1	1165
1800		40	5·1	10	1·3	50	6·4	783
1820		11	1·4	5	0·6	16	2·1	800
1840		35	3·2	3	0·3	38	3·5	1104
1806	Nottingham General[28]*	60	3·9	10	0·7	70	4·6	1522
1837	Radcliffe Infirmary Oxford	10	5	No record		15	7·5	200

Sources: Records of Bristol Royal Infirmary. Bristol Records Office, The Council House, Bristol. Records of the Radcliffe Infirmary. Archives: Oxfordshire Area Health Authority (Teaching), Oxford.
*Inpatient admissions are included.

Role of Epidemiology: Evidence Regarding Burden of Chlorosis

Overall, there is a dearth of statistical or epidemiological evidence about the prevalence of chlorosis. The existing literature shows that the cases of chlorosis were reported from London, Italy, Spain, Europe, and the United States of America (Siddall, 1982). Since it was the pre-epidemiology era, no population-based studies were conducted or reported in the literature (Simon, 1897). Hence, the most important evidence on the burden of chlorosis only comes from the records of the hospitals and dispensaries (Loudon, 1980). The hospital-based data reveals that chlorosis was common among the indigents during the latter half of the eighteenth and throughout the nineteenth centuries. For instance, dispensary records, which are particularly considered valuable sources on the morbidity patterns during the initial industrial revolution, come from the Finsbury Dispensary in London for the year 1800 as shown in Table I (I. S. Loudon, 1980). The dispensary record of one month indicates that amenorrhea and chlorosis were more prevalent conditions as compared to other diseases. Furthermore, in the 12 monthly reports for 1800, out of 3001 admissions at the Finsbury Dispensary, 184 (6.1 %) patients were admitted with chlorosis, which was found to be the third or fourth most common disorder (Loudon, 1980).

The evidence regarding incidence is further summarized in Table II and III which shows that disease was more common across London and in different provinces during late 18th and early 19th centuries (Loudon, 1980).

In addition to this, the records in hospitals were also maintained by age strata as shown in the table IV which depicts that disease was more commonly found among 15 to 24 years' older women as compared to extremes of the age strata (I. S. Loudon, 1980).

Moreover, the existing literature indicates that different physicians have counted and reviewed cases of chlorosis, who either visited outpatient departments or were admitted in the hospitals. For

TABLE IV—*Age-incidence of cases of chlorosis and amenorrhea and of cases of menorrhagia at outpatients department at Bristol Royal Infirmary*

			Age groups			
	10-14	15-24	25-34	35-44	45-54	Total
Amenorrhea and chlorosis						
1760	1	35	22	4	1	63
1800	1	33	6			40
1840	1	26	7	1		35
Menorrhagia						
1760		1	5	6	2	14
1800			3	4	3	10
1840			2	1		3

Source: Outpatient registers, Bristol Royal Infirmary, Bristol Records Office, The Council House, Bristol.

example, in 1836, Dr. Samuel Ashwell described fifteen cases of chlorosis characterized by anemia in young girls, along with menstrual irregularity and other gastrointestinal or pulmonary disorders (Ashwell, 1855). He also mentioned that these chlorotic cases are characterized by reduced appetite and inadequate diet (Ashwell, 1836). Similarly, Dr. Noorden, after reviewing 217 cases in 1905, mentioned that a substantial number of chlorotic cases arise in the same family. Dr. Noorden also highlighted that in addition to symptoms resembling anemia, a considerable number of young women present with loss of appetite, epigastric pain, vomiting, and constipation (King, 2004).

Furthermore, in 1923, Dr. Campbell reviewed the symptomatology of 104 cases that visited in London between 1888 and 1922 (Campbell, 1923). His description of the disease matched with Dr. Noorden's narratives but he also pointed out that a considerable number of cases had low gastric acidity with symptoms persisted for many years (Campbell, 1923).

Role of Iron in Re-conceptualizing Chlorosis to Iron Deficiency Anemia: A Paradigm Shift

Iron was prescribed for almost three centuries for chlorosis indicating that its therapeutic use is far older than the rational explanation of its mode of action, and beliefs regarding its worth have transformed significantly with the passage of time (Haden, 1938). Only recently clinicians have come to know about the effective preparations and ways of administering iron in adequate dosages (Conrad, 2002). Physicians have used iron salts for different purposes since the time of Hippocrates (Haden, 1938). The main tribute for introducing iron to treat chlorosis can be contributed to Dr. Thomas Sydenham, who did not know the mode of action (Sydenham & Latham, 1850). The applications of iron in the earlier years were more often symbolic, with the notion that iron was suggestive of strength and power (Sydenham & Latham, 1850). Thus, for around next 150 years' iron continued to be used for the treatment of chlorosis but with variable results and without a suitable mechanism of action (Haden, 1938; Poskitt, 2003).

It was the French physician, Dr. Pierre Blaud, who first featured the specific action of iron to treat chlorosis and recommended appropriate doses of iron therapy (Fitz, 1937). Dr. Pierre Blaud introduced pills having mixture of ferrous sulfate and potassium carbonate (Neuroth & Lee, 1941). During 1830s, Dr. Blaud prescribed iron in proper dosages even before the estimation of hemoglobin or red blood count (Haden, 1938). Dr. Blaud thought that chlorosis was due to the defective formation of blood, which makes blood an imperfect fluid (Haden, 1938). He further elaborated that chlorotic girls lose the coloring matter in the blood, which is required for stimulating and maintaining the regular functions of the body (Haden, 1938). He also explained that iron medications help blood to restore the most important principle (its coloring substance), which is lost during menstruation (Haden, 1938).

Dr. Blaud suggested the use of a combination of iron sulfate with potassium carbonate because he believed that potassium carbonate increased the absorption of iron (Hudson, 1977). Dr. Blaud initially provided treatment to thirty patients, who were cured and recovered from chlorosis within ten to thirty-two days (Haden, 1938). Dr. Blaud mentioned. however, that iron was used by many physicians in the past but previous failures were due to the use of small and inadequate iron doses (Haden, 1938). Thus, Dr. Blaud emphasized that his promising results were due to the use of the iron preparation he suggested and the large doses of iron he prescribed. For instance, his way of prescribing iron in proper and correct doses is given in the image (Haden, 1938). Dr. Blaud suggested that the success of his prescription was due to the finely divided state of the ferrous salts and the addition of potassium carbonate (Neuroth & Lee, 1941). Moreover, he emphasized the two important principles of iron therapy, the use of ferrous salt, which is easily absorbed as compared to ferric salts and large doses of iron (Lke & Minot, 1923). For several years physicians followed Dr. Blaud's important principles of iron therapy. In fact, the most recent development in iron therapy was also based on the greater strength of ferrous salts and adequate doses of iron (Conrad, 2002).

This prescription gives the equivalent of 5 grains (0.3 Gm.) of ferrous sulfate, or approximately 2 grains (0.1 Gm.) of ferrous carbonate, in each pill.

The method of administration suggested was:

1, 2, 3 day   one pill before breakfast and at bedtime.
4, 5, 6 day   one pill three times a day
7, 8, 9 day   two pills in the morning and evening
10, 11, 12 day two pills three times a day
13, 14, 15 day three pills twice a day
16 and follow-
ing days   four pills three times a day

Role of Hematology in Re-conceptualizing Disease to Iron Deficiency Anemia: A Paradigm Shift

During the mid of 19th century (1852), the first red cell count was made. This was followed by an invention of the first haemoglobinometer in 1876, which resulted in the inception of clinical hematology (Robb-Smith, 1933). Although propositions that the blood might be altered in chlorosis were made as early as 1830, the theory of anemia was only accepted around forty or fifty years later (Loudon, 1980). E. Lloyd Jones, a pathology instructor at Cambridge and a research scholar for the British Medical Association, proposed an explanation of the causes of chlorosis that reflected new research techniques and insights from the science of hematology (Jones, 1897). Jones argued that chlorosis was best understood in relation to the blood changes, mainly a drop in specific blood gravity among young females at puberty (Jones, 1897).

Jones highlighted that there is a significant drop in the specific gravity of blood among chlorotic young females at the age of puberty as compared to males (Jones, 1897). Jones further explained this gender disparity in the drop of blood gravity by using the centrifugal method (revolving tubes of blood at a speed of 1,000 rpm) (Jones, 1897). He found a reduction in the amount of hemoglobin, a less number of red blood cells, and an increase in the proportion of serum to red blood cells in chlorotic girls as compared to males (Jones, 1897).

In 1890s, Dr. Ralph Stockman, physician and lecturer in Edinburgh, wrote/discovered that inorganic iron was utilized to synthesize hemoglobin (Stockman, 1895). He further explained that scientists seeking to cure disease through other methods did not realize that the absence of a small element such as iron could be a cause of disease (Stockman, 1895). Dr. Stockman analyzed the food consumed by chlorotic patients and based on his analyses of iron in different food articles, he found that diet of chlorotic patients contained significantly fewer levels of iron as compared to healthy subjects (Stockman, 1895). More specifically, he demonstrated that the dietary intake of iron of chlorotic patients had 1.3-3.0 mg of iron per day as compared to 6-11 mg of iron found in the diets of healthy subjects (Stockman, 1895). He further explained that onset of menstruation, while the body is actively growing, makes a great demand on the blood (Stockman, 1893). He took advantage of clinical hematology and described that during a menstrual period in a chlorotic girl, the red blood cells fell as much as 10 to 20 percent of their total number. For example, in five days he found that they fell from 4,432,000 to 3,764,000 per cubic millimeter (Stockman, 1895).

Dr. Stockman further highlighted that in chlorotic girls, the decreased red blood cell forming power was due to lack of iron and possibly also to a general impairment of nutritional activity (Stockman, 1893). He emphasized that as soon as iron is given under favorable hygienic conditions, new red blood cells are formed rapidly (Stockman, 1893). Furthermore, he explained that the healthy woman has sufficient reserves of iron in the liver and spleen, but in girls malnourished from any cause including hemorrhage, there is little or no iron in the body to draw on for the production of red cells thus resulting in anemia (Stockman, 1895).

Dr. Stockman also gave a rationale for finding chlorosis more commonly in women as compared to men (Stockman, 1895). He suggested that women generally have about 10 % fewer red blood cells, 8 to 10 % less hemoglobin, and 4 or 5 % more water in the blood as compared to men (Stockman, 1895). Blood of females is, therefore, less able to resist any drain on it mainly during hemorrhage (menstruation). Therefore, it is particularly noticed immediately at puberty when there is greater drain that takes place in young women (Stockman, 1895).

He further emphasized that in 63 cases of chlorosis treated in the hospital, the majority of the cases' red blood cells were lacking in hemoglobin and usually in number, but often many red blood cells were ill-formed and small (Stockman, 1895). Thus the severity of the clinical symptoms depended primarily on the degree of reduction in hemoglobin (Stockman, 1895).
He further explained that in healthy women, 100 cubic centimeters (c.cm) blood yield 21 to 24 c.cm of oxygen, while in chlorotic women the same amount of blood gives only 10 to 15 c.cm of oxygen (Stockman, 1895). Thus, it is the deficiency of hemoglobin, combined with the resultant oxygen deficiency, which gives forms the clinical picture of chlorosis (Stockman, 1895). Hence, Dr. Stockman concluded that there are two main direct causes of chlorosis:blood loss and insufficient supply of iron by the food thatincreases demands for iron (Stockman, 1895).

Combined Role of Hematology and Iron Therapy

The role of iron therapy and development in hematology helped physicians in assessing hemoglobin levels and provide treatment based on the levels of hemoglobin rather than symptoms and gender (Patek & Heath, 1936). For instance, Dr. J Patek gave a detailed account of four chlorotic patients (15 to 16-year-old girls) who were admitted in the hospital during 1930s (Patek & Heath, 1936). He did a thorough analysis of these chlorotic girls by taking detailed history, measured their growth, examined their blood for hemoglobin and iron, stool for occult blood, and conducted a gastric analysis (Patek & Heath, 1936). After taking detailed history and undertaking detailed analysis, Dr. Patek analyzed factors responsible for iron deficiency in these adolescent girls (Patek & Heath, 1936). He found that these girls did not have enough iron in their diet. The total iron found in their diet was 5.4 mg, which could only satisfy the maintenance needs of this patient, but could not efficiently make up the hemoglobin deficit (Patek & Heath, 1936). Furthermore, Dr. Patek found that mothers of these girls were iron deficient during their pregnancy; as a result, sufficient iron stores failed to transfer from mother to these girls, thus making them susceptible to iron deficiency anemia (Patek & Heath, 1936). Moreover, Dr. Patek also highlighted that gastric analysis of these girls showed less acid in the stomach of these patients(adequate amount of acid is important for iron absorption) (Patek & Heath, 1936).

Dr. Patek treated these cases with adequate iron therapy and observed a prompt recovery in these girls. Specifically, he saw hemoglobin levels rise from 40 to 81 percent in two months (Patek & Heath, 1936). With his analysis, Dr. Patek made the conclusion that chlorosis had not disappeared; rather, it was prevalent in the form of iron deficiency anemia (Patek & Heath, 1936). He further said that chlorosis is the exaggeration of a normal tendency towards anemia in adolescent girls, created by the increased demand for iron made by growth and by menstrual blood loss (Patek & Heath, 1936). Changes in diet and nutrition after 1900, along with an increased understanding of ovarian function and iron deficiency anemia, provide some explanation of the disease's reconceptualization to iron deficiency anemia by 1930 (Brumberg, 1982). Although now generally rare in the population, recently, a 9-year-old Filipino decent girl was diagnosed with symptoms of chlorosis and severe deficiency of iron. The girl was successfully treated and her symptoms disappeared with iron salt therapy (Perdahl-Wallace & Schwartz, 2006).

Conclusion

Chlorosis was an important subject of medical literature until the second to third decades of twentieth century. The hematology and iron therapy has played an important role in re-conceptualizing disease from Chlorosis to iron deficiency anemia. In addition, overall improvement in nutrition, the environment of the working class and intake of adequate diet have also contributed. This disease has not disappeared from the world; rather, it is prevalent as one of the most common types of anemia (i.e. iron deficiency anemia in the contemporary world affecting most of women of reproductive age, children and adults mainly in the developing countries).

References

Ashwell, S. (1836). Observations on chlorosis and its complications. Guy's Hospital Reports, 1, 529.

Ashwell, S. (1855). A practical treatise on the diseases peculiar to women: Blanchard and Lea.

Brumberg, J. J. (1982). Chlorotic girls, 1870-1920: A historical perspective on female adolescence. *Child Development*, 1468-1477.

Campbell, J. (1923). Chlorosis, a study of the Guy's Hospital cases during the last thirty years, with some remarks on its etiology and the causes of its diminished frequency. Guy's Hospital Reports, 73, 247-297.

Christian, H. A. (1903). A Sketch of the History of the Treatment of Chlorosis with Iron. *Medical library and historical journal, 1*(3), 176.

Conrad, M. E. (2002). Iron deficiency anemia. *Medicine Journal, 3*, 114-124.

Comrie, J. D. (1922) Selected Works of Thomas Sydenham, p. 132. Bale Sons &. Danielson,. London, England

Fitz, R. (1937). The Whole Story of Clinical Research in a Nutshell. *Canadian Medical Association Journal, 37*(2), 182.

Guggenheim, K. Y. (1995). Chlorosis: the rise and disappearance of a nutritional disease. *The Journal of*

nutrition, *125*(7), 1822-1825.

Haden, R. L. (1938). Historical Aspects of Iron Therapy In Anemia: Chairman's Address. *Journal of the American Medical Association, 111*(12), 1059-1061.

Hudson, R. P. (1977). The biography of disease: lessons from chlorosis. *Bulletin of the History of Medicine, 51*(3), 448.

Jones, E. L. (1897). Chlorosis: special anemia of young women: causes, pathology, and treatment: being a report to the scientific grants committee of the British Medical Association: Baillière, Tindall & Cox.

King, H. (2004). The disease of virgins: green sickness, chlorosis and the problems of puberty: Routledge.

Lke, r. I., & Minot, g. R. (1923). Chapter iv chlorosis. Nelson Loose-leaf Living Medicine, 4, 33.

Loudon, I. (1984). The diseases called chlorosis. Psychological medicine, 14(1), 27-36.

Loudon, I. S. (1980). Chlorosis, anemia, and anorexia nervosa. British Medical Journal, 281(6256), 1669.

Major, R. H. (1945). Classic descriptions of disease: with biographical sketches of the authors: Charles C. Thomas Publisher

Mettler, C. (1947) History of Medicine, p. 366. Blakiston, Philadelphia, PA.

Neuroth, M., & Lee, C. (1941). A history of Blaud's pills. Journal of the American Pharmaceutical Association, 30(2), 60-63.

Osler, W. (1892) Principles and Practice of Medicine, 7th Ã©d., pp. 686-696; (1911) pp. 721-731. Appleton & Co., New York, NY.

Patek, A. J., & Heath, C. W. (1936). Chlorosis. Journal of the American Medical Association, 106(17), 1463-1466.

Perdahl-Wallace, E., & Schwartz, R. H. (2006). A girl with green complexion and iron deficiency: Chlorosis revisited. Clinical pediatrics, 45(2), 187-189.

Poskitt, E. M. (2003). Early history of iron deficiency. British journal of haematology, 122(4), 554-562.

Rand, R. (1986). Hysteron Proteron, or 'Woman First'. Oxford Literary Review, 8(1), 51-56.

Robb-Smith, A. (1933). The history of the hedgehog's rosary. St Bartholomew's Hosp J, 40, 149-152.

Siddall, A. C. (1982). Chlorosis-etiology reconsidered. Bulletin of the History of Medicine, 56(2), 254.

Simon, C. E. (1897). A Study of Thirty-One Cases of Chlorosis, With Special Reference To The Etiology And The Dietrtic Treatment of The Disease. The American Journal of the Medical Sciences (1827-1924), 113(4), 399.

Starobinski, J. (1981). Chlorosis–the 'green sickness'. *Psychological medicine, 11*(3), 459-468.

Sydenham, T. (1718) Whole Works, p. 321. Browne, London, England.

Stockman, R. (1893). The treatment of chlorosis by iron and some other drugs. British Medical Journal, 1(1687), 881.

Stockman, R. (1895). Observations on the causes and treatment of chlorosis. British Medical Journal, 2(1824), 1473.

Sydenham, T., & Latham, R. G. (1850). The Works of Thomas Sydenham, MD (Vol. 2): Printed for the Sydenham Society.

Taylor, F., Bramwell, B., Williamson, R., Clarke, J. M., Gairdner, T., Affleck, J., . . . Ransom, W. (1896). A discussion on anaemia: its causation, varieties, associated pathology, and treatment. The British Medical Journal, 719-728.

Zilborg, G. & Henry, G. H. (1947) A History of Medical Psychology,47. Norton, New York, NY.

Chapter 2: An overview of anemia, its associated factors and adverse outcomes among women of reproductive age

Anemia and its associated adverse outcomes

Anemia is one of the major public health issues among women of reproductive age (WRA), as it leads to high maternal and infant morbidity and mortality (1). Anemia occurs when the number and size of red blood cells or the hemoglobin (Hb) concentration fall below an established cut-off value, consequently impairing the capacity of the blood to transport oxygen to the body (2, 3). The World Health Organization (WHO) defines anemia as Hb levels of <12.0 g/dL among women of reproductive age (4).

There is a complex impact of anemia on the health of women and children (5). The consequences of anemia vary according to the type and severity of anemia among WRA (6, 7). Several studies have shown that anemia among pregnant women can result in poor maternal and fetal outcomes such as abortion, intrauterine growth retardation, post-partum hemorrhage, stillbirths, low-birth-weight, prematurity, and perinatal mortality (8-11). For instance, a review of observational studies found a linear association between maternal anemia and maternal mortality, with each 10 g/L increase in maternal hemoglobin associated with a 29% reduction in maternal mortality (12). Likewise, findings from a systematic review revealed that 25% of low birth weight babies, 44% of preterm deliveries, and 21% of perinatal mortality are attributable to anemia during pregnancy in low- and middle-income countries (LMICs) (13). Furthermore, a meta-analysis showed an increased risk of preterm birth among women who experienced anemia in the first trimester with an overall odds ratio of 1.32 (14). Most recently, a study based on the WHO multi-country survey demonstrated that severe anemia is associated with a two-fold increase in the risk of maternal death (15).

Burden of Anemia in developing countries

Although anemia has been shown to affect women in both high and low- and middle-income countries, the major burden of anemia is found in LMICs (16, 17). More specifically, anemia affects nearly two-thirds of WRA in LMICs (18). According to the WHO, about half a billion of WRA are anemic worldwide, with a higher burden of anemia in South-East Asia (41.9%), followed by African and Eastern Mediterranean regions (19). For example, studies from India show the prevalence of anemia among WRA ranges from 50% to 90% across different geographic areas of India (20-22). Likewise, community- based cross-sectional studies conducted in Ethiopia demonstrate that 34.5% to 56.8% of the WRA are suffering from anemia across different regions of Ethiopia (23-25). Similarly, one study conducted in Uganda found that 63.1% of women are anemic in Uganda, and one study from Bangladesh revealed that more than a third of women are anemic in Bangladesh (26). In addition, estimates in high-risk populations suggest that total anemia prevalence may be as high as 50% to 80% in developing countries, with as many as 10% to 20% having moderate to severe anemia (27). Although multiple interventions have shown to reduce the prevalence of anemia worldwide by 12% between 1992 and 2011, these efforts did not have a similar impact in LMICs (28).

Factors or predictors of Anemia among women of reproductive age

The existing literature highlights that multiple factors, such as smokeless tobacco, infectious and chronic diseases, and a dietary inadequacy, especially of food sources rich in iron, folic acid, and vitamin B12 can cause anemia among WRA mainly in developing countries (29-31). In addition, studies conducted in different developing countries have shown that normal physiological changes of pregnancy, hemoglobinopathies, malaria, HIV, and hookworm infestation can also contribute to anemia among WRA in developing countries (30, 32, 33). Additional factors that predispose WRA to anemia include differences in lifestyles, socio-demographic factors, hygiene conditions, and genetic susceptibility (34, 35). These factors can be broadly classified as below:
   1. **Socio-demographic factors**

Socio-demographic factors included women's age, education, parity, current pregnancy status, interpregnancy interval, place of residence, socioeconomic status and religion. Two studies reported women's age to be an important determinant of anemia (Table 2) and with older women more likely to experience anemia(1, 2). Four studies found that women's education was an important determinant of anemia, all of which demonstrated illiterate women were more likely to be anemic as compared to their counterparts (1-4). Likewise, four studies found strong associations between parity and anemia as shown in Table 2. Higher parity with more than three children was found to be positively associated with anemia as compared to the nulliparous women among all reviewed studies (4-7).

Two studies found a strong positive association between a small inter-pregnancy interval of less than 1 year and anemia (Table 2) (3, 8). Six studies showed pregnancy as an important risk factor for anemia with more women found to be anemic in the second and third trimester as compared to the first trimester(4, 5, 7, 9-11). In addition, three studies indicated that socioeconomic status played a significant role in anemia and that being poor was found to be a determinant of anemia (1, 2, 12). In addition, two studies found a positive and significant association between place of residence and anemia(2, 9). Lastly, one study found that non-Muslims were more at risk for anemia as compared to Muslims(1).

2. **Nutrition-related factors**

Most of the studies assessed nutritional factors through bio-markers such as serum iron, folic acid, and serum ferritin. However, some of the studies also assessed nutritional status based on the intake of foods and body mass index (BMI) of the women. Thus nutrition-related factors included iron deficiency, folic acid deficiency, serum ferritin levels, consumption of eggs and tea, consumption of fruits, history of pica (clay, dirt, or ice) and history of breastfeeding.

Three studies found iron and folic acid deficiency as important factors for anemia, demonstrating iron deficient and folic acid-deficient women were more likely to be anemic as compared to their counterparts(7, 8, 13). Moreover, two studies found undernourishment (BMI of < 18.5kg/m^2) as a significant positive factor for anemia(6). Likewise, one study found that a history of pica was strongly associated with anemia with an adjusted odds ratio (OR) of 3.7(10). Similarly; one study conducted in Ethiopia showed Chewing Khat (chewable tobacco) was also positively associated with anemia(11). Moreover, consumption of fruits/vegetables low in vitamin A was also was associated with anemia in one study conducted in the Democratic Republic of Congo (DRC)(3). One study conducted in Bangladesh indicated breastfeeding as a determinant of anemia among women(1).

3. Co-morbid and other factors

Studies have also assessed important diseases such as malaria, hookworm infestation and chronic illness as factors contributing to anemia. For example, three studies assessed the association between malaria and anemia and two of these found positive significant association, with ORs ranging from 2.06 to 11.19(3, 6). In contrast, one of these studies,conducted in Uganda, found an inverse relationship(12). Similarly, hookworm infestations were positively associated with anemia (OR: 2.37) in studies conducted in Kenya and Ethiopia(6, 9). History of chronic illness was associated with anemia in one study conducted in Ethiopia, with an OR of 1.11(13). Additionally, other factors such as biomass fuel usage, current usage of contraceptive methods and usage of ITN (Insecticide-treated nets) were also positively associated with anemia (1, 5, 9).

Burden of Anemia in Pakistan

Like other LMICs, anemia is common in Pakistan. For example, literature shows that around 75% of WRA are anemic in rural areas of Pakistan (34). In addition, a recently conducted national nutritional survey in Pakistan demonstrates that 41.7% of WRA are anemic in Pakistan(36). The same survey also highlights women in rural areas (44.3%) are more anemic when compared to urban areas (40.2%) of Pakistan (36). More specifically, iron deficiency anemia is more prevalent in Pakistan than developed countries and 18.2% of WRA are iron deficient, which is more noticeable in rural areas (18.7%) than urban areas (17.4%) (36). The province of Sindh has the highest proportion of iron deficiency anemia (23.8%), followed by Balochistan (19.0%) and Punjab (18.7%) (36). Similarly, another study conducted in one of Pakistan's rural areas shows that 77.0% of Pakistani women are anemic; of this, 20.8 % of the women are mildly anemic and 56.5% of the women suffer from moderate to severe anemia (37). Thus anemia is more prevalent in the rural areas of Pakistan, where it isoften severe and is linked to adverse health consequences (37). For example, this study also reveals that rural Pakistani women who are severely anemic are more likely to experience postpartum hemorrhage, intrauterine growth retardation, stillbirths, preterm births, and low birth weight babies (37).

In addition, very few studies conducted in the urban areas of Pakistan have explored determinants of anemia among urban WRA (38-40). These studies have found that urban Pakistani women who are not educated, belong to poor socioeconomic status, have given birth to more thanfour children, who consume a large amount of tea, have a history of pica (eating non-nutritious substances:

fuller's earth, clay or ice), who have food insecurity, and consume diet inadequate in iron and folic acid are more likely to be anemic when compared to their counterparts in the urban areas (38-40). Although these studies have investigated the determinants of anemia in Pakistan, there are certain gaps that need to be addressed (38-40). Firstly, existing studies are mainly focused on large urban areas of Pakistan rather than rural areas where the burden of anemia is higher. In addition, there are differences in the socio-demographic, cultural, economic, and dietary factors between rural and urban areas, which do not accurately characterize anemia in a rural setting (41). Therefore, studies of urban populations may not be relevant in the rural context of Pakistan. Secondly, anemia is a complex and multifactorial phenomenon that should be understood holistically. Current studies in urban settings provide important insights about sociodemographic and reproductive determinants, but leave key biological and dietary determinants unaddressed and therefore, poorly understood (38-40). Lastly, investigators in the urban studies have not utilized objective measurements of biological factors (e.g: serum iron, ferritin, serum B12, and folic acid, a malarial parasite in the blood, etc.) in the blood. Rather, their results are based on self-reported data, which is subjective and may have produced biased estimates of associations between biological determinants and anemia among WRA.

Although studies have provided limited evidence on the burden and adverse outcomes of anemia among WRA in rural Pakistan, there is a major gap regarding the prevalence and determinants of anemia mainly in rural Pakistan. Because anemia is a common medical condition affecting maternal and child health in Pakistan, understanding the determinants of anemia among WRA is of paramount importance. Thus, it is crucial to know why rural Pakistani WRA are anemic and what are the determinants of anemia among rural WRA in Pakistan? More specifically, there is a need to investigate the underlying determinants of anemia comprehensively across the range of socio-demographic, reproductive, dietary and biological domains in rural Pakistan, which have not been previously studied in this context. Understanding these determinants holistically will enable the development of local strategies and targeted interventions to address the anemia's burden among WRA in rural Pakistan.

References

1. Milman N. Anemia—still a major health problem in many parts of the world! Annals of hematology. 2011;90(4):369-77.
2. Beutler E, Waalen J. The definition of anemia: what is the lower limit of normal of the blood hemoglobin concentration? Blood. 2006;107(5):1747-50.
3. Cappellini MD, Motta I, editors. Anemia in clinical practice—definition and classification: does hemoglobin change with aging? Seminars in hematology; 2015: Elsevier.
4. Organization WH. Haemoglobin concentrations for the diagnosis of anaemia and assessment of severity. World Health Organization; 2011.
5. Allen LH. Anemia and iron deficiency: effects on pregnancy outcome. The American journal of clinical nutrition. 2000;71(5):1280S-4S.
6. Kalaivani K. Prevalence & consequences of anaemia in pregnancy. Indian J Med Res.

2009;130(5):627-33.

7.   Kozuki N, Lee A, Katz J. Child Health Epidemiology Reference G. Moderate to severe, but not mild, maternal anemia is associated with increased risk of small-for-gestational-age outcomes. J Nutr. 2012;142(2):358-62.

8.   Beckert RH, Baer RJ, Anderson JG, Jelliffe-Pawlowski LL, Rogers EE. Maternal anemia and pregnancy outcomes: a population-based study. Journal of Perinatology. 2019:1.

9.   Hare GM, Freedman J, Mazer CD. risks of anemia and related management strategies: can perioperative blood management improve patient safety? Canadian Journal of Anesthesia/Journal canadien d'anesthésie. 2013;60(2):168-75.

10.   Kavle JA, Stoltzfus RJ, Witter F, Tielsch JM, Khalfan SS, Caulfield LE. Association between anaemia during pregnancy and blood loss at and after delivery among women with vaginal births in Pemba Island, Zanzibar, Tanzania. Journal of health, population, and nutrition. 2008;26(2):232.

11.   Tunkyi K, Moodley J. Anemia and pregnancy outcomes: a longitudinal study. The Journal of Maternal-Fetal & Neonatal Medicine. 2018;31(19):2594-8.

12.   Black RE, Victora CG, Walker SP, Bhutta ZA, Christian P, De Onis M, et al. Maternal and child undernutrition and overweight in low-income and middle-income countries. The lancet. 2013;382(9890):427-51.

13.   Rahman MM, Abe SK, Rahman MS, Kanda M, Narita S, Bilano V, et al. Maternal anemia and risk of adverse birth and health outcomes in low-and middle-income countries: systematic review and meta-analysis, 2. The American journal of clinical nutrition. 2016;103(2):495-504.

14.   Xiong X, Buekens P, Alexander S, Demianczuk N, Wollast E. Anemia during pregnancy and birth outcome: a meta-analysis. American journal of perinatology. 2000;17(03):137-46.

15.   Daru J, Zamora J, Fernández-Félix BM, Vogel J, Oladapo OT, Morisaki N, et al. Risk of maternal mortality in women with severe anaemia during pregnancy and post partum: a multilevel analysis. The Lancet Global Health. 2018;6(5):e548-e54.

16.   Organization WH. The global prevalence of anaemia in 2011. Geneva: World Health Organization; 2015. 2017.

17.   Sifakis S, Pharmakides G. Anemia in pregnancy. Annals of the New York Academy of Sciences. 2000;900(1):125-36.

18.   Ouédraogo S, Koura GK, Bodeau-Livinec F, Accrombessi MM, Massougbodji A, Cot M. Maternal anemia in pregnancy: assessing the effect of routine preventive measures in a malaria- endemic area. The American journal of tropical medicine and hygiene. 2013;88(2):292-300.

19.   Organization WH. The global prevalence of anaemia in 2011. The global prevalence of anaemia in 20112015.

20.   Bentley M, Griffiths P. The burden of anemia among women in India. European journal of clinical nutrition. 2003;57(1):52-60.

21.   Panja TK, Sinha NK, Chakrabortty S, Maiti S, Dutta D, Kundu P, et al. Prevalence of

anaemia in varied nutritional state among the women of reproductive ages belonging to low socioeconomic status of rural India. Age (year). 2019;29(9.88):28.70-30.27.

22.   Panyang R, Teli AB, Saikia SP. Prevalence of anemia among the women of childbearing age belonging to the tea garden community of Assam, India: A community-based study. Journal of family medicine and primary care. 2018;7(4):734.

23.   Addis Alene K, Mohamed Dohe A. Prevalence of anemia and associated factors among pregnant women in an urban area of Eastern Ethiopia. Anemia. 2014;2014.

24.   Getachew M, Yewhalaw D, Tafess K, Getachew Y, Zeynudin A. Anaemia and associated risk factors among pregnant women in Gilgel Gibe dam area, Southwest Ethiopia. Parasites & vectors. 2012;5(1):296.

25.   Haidar J. Prevalence of anaemia, deficiencies of iron and folic acid and their determinants in Ethiopian women. Journal of health, population, and nutrition. 2010;28(4):359.

26.   Chowdhury HA, Ahmed KR, Jebunessa F, Akter J, Hossain S, Shahjahan M. Factors associated with maternal anaemia among pregnant women in Dhaka city. BMC women's health. 2015;15(1):77.

27.   Organization WH. The prevalence of anaemia in women: a tabulation of available information. World Health Organization; 1992.

28.   Organization WH. Global nutrition targets 2025: Breastfeeding policy brief. World Health Organization; 2014.

29.   Zhang SM, Willett WC, Selhub J, Hunter DJ, Giovannucci EL, Holmes MD, et al. Plasma folate, vitamin B6, vitamin B12, homocysteine, and risk of breast cancer. Journal of the National Cancer Institute. 2003;95(5):373-80.

30.   Velikkakam T, Fiuza JA, Gaze ST. Overview of hookworm infection in humans. Neglected Tropical Diseases-South Asia: Springer; 2017. p. 121-35.

31.   Shedge H, Kulkarni S. Maternal Smokeless Tobacco Use in Pregnancy and Adverse Health Outcomes in Newborn Babies (LBW): A Systematic Review. Asian Man (The)-An International Journal. 2017;11(2):180-2.

32.   Anchang-Kimbi JK, Nkweti VN, Ntonifor HN, Apinjoh TO, Chi HF, Tata RB, et al. Profile of red blood cell morphologies and causes of anaemia among pregnant women at first clinic visit in the mount Cameroon area: a prospective cross sectional study. BMC research notes. 2017;10(1):645.

33.   Inamdar AS, Croucher RE, Chokhandre MK, Mashyakhy MH, Marinho VC. Maternal smokeless tobacco use in pregnancy and adverse health outcomes in newborns: a systematic review. Nicotine & Tobacco Research. 2014;17(9):1058-66.

34.   Baig-Ansari N, Badruddin SH, Karmaliani R, Harris H, Jehan I, Pasha O, et al. Anemia prevalence and risk factors in pregnant women in an urban area of Pakistan. Food and nutrition bulletin. 2008;29(2):132-9.

35.   Ismail IM, Kahkashan A, Antony A, Sobhith V. Role of socio-demographic and cultural factors on anemia in a tribal population of North Kerala, India. International journal of community medicine and public health. 2017;3(5):1183-8.

36.   Ministry of National Services Regulation and Coordination (MoNHSR&C) GoP. National Nutrition Survey. 2018.

37.   Parks S, Hoffman MK, Goudar SS, Patel A, Saleem S, Ali SA, et al. Maternal anaemia and maternal, fetal, and neonatal outcomes in a prospective cohort study in India and Pakistan. BJOG: An International Journal of Obstetrics & Gynaecology. 2018.

38.   Ullah I, Zahid M, Khan MI, Shah M. Prevalence of anemia in pregnant women in district Karak, Khyber Pakhtunkhwa, Pakistan. International Journal of Biosciences. 2013;3:77-83.

39.   Anjum A, Manzoor M, Manzoor N, Shakir HA. Prevalence of anemia during pregnancy in district Faisalabad, Pakistan. Punjab Univ J Zool. 2015;30(1):15-20.

40.   Habib MA, Raynes-Greenow C, Soofi SB, Ali N, Nausheen S, Ahmed I, et al. Prevalence and determinants of iron deficiency anemia among non-pregnant women of reproductive age in Pakistan. Asia Pacific journal of clinical nutrition. 2018;27(1):195.

Chapter 3: Perceptions of the community of rural Pakistan about nutrition and anemia

This chapter gives an overview of the perceptions and beliefs of rural community people and health care providers about anemia among women of reproductive age. A group of women, men, and health care providers were interviewed in one of the rural communities of Pakistan to know their perceptions, ideas, opinions, knowledge, and practices about anemia.

Knowledge of rural community about Nutrition

During the interviews, most of the males reported that nutrition means good or proper and hygienic food on time and if we eat good food, it will make us healthy. There are various sources of good nutrition such as vegetables, fish, chicken, fruits, lassi, butter, milk. More specifically, fish and beef contain a huge amount of energy. Few males also mentioned that usually rich people eat good and healthy food such as fish and beef while poor people eat pulses (daal) and vegetables (sabzi). For instance, rich people eat three meals a day; but poor people are unable to eat complete meals. In addition, few males also emphasized that in our area, we usually do not get pure food and good water. Females of the community verbalized that fruits such as apple, banana, and pomegranate, and vegetables including spinach, cauliflower and ladyfinger, Brinjal, ridge gourd and comprise food. Juices are also good but they are useful for a temporary period because juices contain chemicals.

"We belong to Sindhi culture so mostly we eat fish rather than eating vegetables and meat" (Female of the community)".

The majority of the women did not know about anemia and few verbalized that deficiency of blood in the body is labeled as anemia or anemia means women are weak. Females also mentioned in the interview that anemia is not a good thing and it means one needs to take treatment from doctor or blood transfusion as per the advice of health care provider. They also verbalized that blood is synthesized from food and water and when we eat 10 grams of food then body forms 1 drop of blood. Likewise, most of the males also iterated that we don't have that much information about anemia but we can have an idea from the physical appearance of woman as she will appear weak in case of blood deficiency. One of the males mentioned that women don't have the awareness that we are getting weak and we need to consult the doctor. In rural areas, women are not educated enough so they don't take care of themselves properly.

According to health care providers, rural women consider blood deficiency as a normal process of the delivery process. They think that these are usual symptoms, which appear during each delivery they undergo. According to females, their elders have told us that this is not a disease rather this is a normal process, which happens during delivery and even we (elderly female) had given birth to 8 children but we are healthy.

"Women think that blood deficiency is a normal process which happens during delivery and their elderly females tell them that this is not a disease or health problem"(Health care provider)

Health Seeking Behavior of rural women

The healthcare providers of the study believed that every woman who visits the clinic to receive ANC services is being counseled for eating healthy and iron-rich food. However, even after counseling, women remain addicted to chewable tobacco [ghutka/mawa/chura in local language] and continue to consume harmful substances because of poor health-seeking behaviors. Few health providers indicated that they also prescribe medicine when women are severely anemic; however, women do not adhere to prescribed medicines due to financial constraints and poor health-seeking behaviors. Few health care providers also mentioned that women do not take care of their health unless they are properly counseled. They highlighted that usually women visit clinics during 2nd trimester, with hemoglobin (Hb) levels of 6 to 7gm/dl, and we give them parental iron to help them survive till the time of delivery. In addition, women do not follow the recommended number of antenatal visits or 3 to 4 investigations endorsed by the World Health organization during antenatal care. Moreover, during 1st trimester, women refuse to go for any investigation and it becomes difficult for us to do their assessment and diagnose any particular health problem. Health care providers also emphasized that usually women visit late in the last month of pregnancy and we ask them where were you throughout the pregnancy and usually they are silent and do not have any answer. Secondly, females also do not revisit after they deliver their child, and 4 out of 10 hardly revisit. What are their conditions, how they are living, and what types of problems they face we are not aware because she does not come back after delivery?
On the other hand, females mentioned that when we go to hospitals, doctors don't give us proper time and attention. They just try to increase their number of patients and see one patient for a few minutes and call the others.

"During antennal care women usually prefer to get their Ultrasound done to identify the sex of the baby rather than health of their child" (HCP, IDI- 01)

On the other hand, women of the community verbalized that they do not have enough money to purchase healthy food items and therefore they continue to eat whatever is available at home and in the fields. While men of the community reported that women do not take care of themselves as they lift heavy weights and continue to consume chewable tobacco the whole day. In addition, few males also highlighted that women carry their children in their womb for nine months without having proper checkups during pregnancy due to lack of money. Furthermore, men also verbalized

22

that we are least bothered for our health and we think that life will move on without putting any further efforts to improve health. If someone gets sick he or she takes three days to go and see the doctor or seek treatment.

"Everyone is busy in their problems and they don't think about their children and their health issues" (Female of the community)".

Few males mentioned that even though everything is available in a government hospital, medical doctors ask us to come to their private clinics, where they practice in the evening. Since these doctors cost more than the government facilities, we usually avoid visiting them.

"When we go to the government hospital, doctors say that we practice in "Doctors Street" in the evening and your wife should come to visit me in my private clinic where I will perform some tests and start treatment (Females)"

Signs, symptoms, and burden of Anemia

The healthcare providers reported that the community women have clear signs of anemia such as fatigue, pale skin, leg cramps, edema, etc. Doctors further mentioned that we assess conjunctiva of eyes to find out the severity of anemia and then we immediately perform hemoglobin tests to further confirm the severity of anemia so that the treatment can be provided accordingly. Providers mentioned that in lab tests reports their Hemoglobin is usually lower than 8 gm/dl due to frequent pregnancies. Health care providers also highlighted that for every 100 females we assess, almost 60 to 80 females are anemic and if I measure it on a scale of 10, so 8 out of 10 females are anemic. One of the male health care providers highlighted that around 99% of pregnant women are anemic in our area and anemia is more common among males as compared to females.

In addition, women have been found with Hb levels of 3 to 4gm/dl during their pregnancy and low hemoglobin is the most important cause to refer patients to other doctors. On inquiring about anemia symptoms, the women in FDGs verbalized that they have difficulty in performing the routine work due to dizziness and loss of energy, feel tired even after doing small work and they fell due to weakness. They mentioned that we do not have enough energy to move from one place to another. In addition, females also mentioned that they become short of breath, or feel difficulty in breathing, feel shivering, become pale, complain of gastric burning due to anemia. Women also mentioned that they can also identify blood deficiency from the nail buds and the eyes of the woman as eyes become white and women develop holes in their nails. In addition, a group of females highlighted that women usually lie down on the bed due to anemia and become uncomfortable or do not feel good. According to women, due to blood deficiency in the body, eve vision of women gets affected, eyes will become dull and heartbeat also increases. Men of the households reported that due to anemia the color of eyes become white and nails become yellow.

"We generally get an idea of blood deficiency from the hands and eyes of women as they become white. Women feel weak and unable to perform work. Upon checkup, doctors ask for some blood tests and let us know that women are (Male of the community)"

"Due to blood deficiency, our blood pressure also goes down, and we cannot perform any work" (Female of the community)".

Causes and consequences of Anemia

Doctors and health care providers in Pakistan believe that the intake of chewable tobacco [ghutka/mawa/chura in local language] is one of the major causes of anemia among pregnant women. The women in the district have developed an addiction for chewable tobacco (Ghutka) as it damages the mucosal membrane and causes addiction, which has eventually led to poor dietary habits among women, causing iron deficiency. Moreover, Ghutka prevents the absorption of iron thus resulting in anemia. Gutka reduces the appetite of women and they neither eat nor drink water rather keep Ghutka in their mouth for a couple of hours. This prevents them from consuming an adequate diet and they become week and develop anemia or infections.

Females also mentioned that they have more tensions as compared to men. Their husbands are far from home for the whole day or sometimes even a month and usually, women get tensed whenever their children get sick. Our husbands come home like guests but we have to stay at home with our children all the time. These tensions make us more week.

Most men reported that women in rural areas can't take care of themselves even when they are pregnant. They can't get a proper diet and also don't consult with doctors. In addition, men also reported that early marriages also common in rural areas, girls get married soon after puberty which results in many pregnancies and causes anemia. Further, doctors verbalized that people in rural areas don't take anemia as a serious issue, especially male has no awareness about anemia. Alongside, consumption of fuller's earth [multani mud in local language] is also considered as an indirect cause of anemia because women tend to avoid the intake of vegetables and fruits due to such cravings. Additionally, females of the highlighted that strenuous work performed by pregnant women in fields could also be a factor leading to anemia. Beside, illiteracy, lack of awareness about the causes of anemia, and limited antenatal checkups were also reported as main causes of iron deficiency by TBAs and health care providers. Further, working barefoot in the field was also reported as a cause for anemia by one of the TBAs as it might provide a favorable condition to worms to pass from the feet into the body. Additionally, few mothers mentioned that because they are poor, they don't get enough food to eat like poultry, vegetables, and therefore they tend to have this deficiency.

Almost all health care providers iterated that a frequent number of pregnancies is one of the important causes of anemia in our district. Thus females, who do not take enough breaks between pregnancies or those who have a poor diet or unable to take enough food are more anemic. For example, a female having 6 children will either feed herself or her children, and usually, she feeds her children rather than herself. Moreover, they have plenty of work to do such as giving care to their livestock, working in the fields so they do not get time to take care of themselves and become anemic. Secondly, women also breastfeed their children but do not consume the required calories to meet the demands of her body resulting in anemia.

"We are addicted, we will not eat a meal but we will buy gutka even though gutka is expensive than medicines (Male of the community)"

"We are habitual. We love eating Ghutkas" (Female of the community)"

"In Villages women have workload, they work in fields all the time without slippers, I think this is the reason they get blood deficiency. From feet, heat enters the body, which affects their eyes and blood gets dry as well (Health care provider)"

"Those women who are just sitting at home and doing nothing, they are healthy and their blood level is high" (Health care provider)"

"In the present time, the major cause of anemia is frequent pregnancies, every female have almost 9 to 10 children" (Health care provider)"

"GOD knows how many children a woman produces because usually, they do not tell us how many children are alive. I have received a patient who has 23 gravida with six to seven miscarriages. Is this not the reason for being anemic?" (Health care provider)

"Woman feeds one child, works in fields, simultaneously taking another baby in the womb and have inadequate diet will end up having anemia (Health care provider)".

"Here in rural areas early marriages are very common and this is our biggest mistake. We just fix their marriages once they reach puberty. We don't think that are they mature enough to take this responsibility or not. In urban areas, people send their girls to school so that they become aware of everything but here we don't do this (Male of the community)"

Consequences of anemia for women and their children

Consequences for pregnant women
Women verbalized that due to anemia they experience vertigo and weakness, which stop them to actively perform daily routine activities. Some Women voiced that due to iron deficiency, many women have lost their lives either before or after childbirth. Additionally, some females thought

25

that due to blood deficiency, the pregnancy gets complicated, and due to which pregnant women has to undergo a big surgery (Cesarean Section). Women also verbalized that due to blood deficiency, a woman can develop seizures, dehydration, and if the baby is not aborted then bleeding occurs. Health care providers mentioned that anemia can also cause postpartum hemorrhage (PPH). If a woman with HB of 5 gm/dl gives birth to a child, she can end up with severe blood loss and lose more than 500 ml of the blood in a single day and we can estimate that how much will be lost in 40 days' post-partum. The chances of PPH increases if a woman comes to the clinic with HB of 3 to 4gm/dl. In addition to PPH, anemia can cause antepartum hemorrhage and headache among pregnant women.

"If she is anemic and has blood deficiency then she will not be able to deliver the child through normal delivery and she will have to undergo a big surgery, which can result in death. (Female of the community)"

Consequences for children

Women of the rural communities believe that child growth will be affected as a consequence of anemia. In addition, few females highlighted that anemia may cause miscarriage or stillbirth. Other females reported that the child may suffer from premature birth, low-birth weight, congenital anomalies, malnutrition, and convulsions as a consequence of iron-deficiency. Females also verbalized that due to anemia, children will not be able to gain sufficient weight and will develop different diseases.

Males of the communities also voiced their concerns about child growth retardation due to anemia and emphasized that women should have a nutritious diet to avoid such long-term complications. Health care providers mentioned that maternal anemia results in an unhealthy, week, premature, and growth-restarted children.

If proper nutrition is not transferred from mother to the child then the child will become ill (Male)"

"When a mother eats proper diet during pregnancy and takes care of herself, she will deliver a healthy baby" (Female)"

"Child may die in the mother's womb due to blood deficiency in woman' (Female)"

Whom to contact?

Females of the community also mentioned that pregnancy care is usually received by TBAs and doctors. In addition, few women reported that in an emergency, pregnant women are referred to the public (Civil hospital) and private facilities for pregnancy care and childbirth. Women in the rural areas mentioned that as an initial step they are being examined by TBAs who help them to visit doctors if required. Females also took names of different health care providers whom they visit either in the government or private hospitals. Females said that they also visit doctors of their village whom they call as Baji (big sister) and take medicines from her. Some of the females said that we usually take care of ourselves at home and do not visit the doctor.

We also perform different totkas (home remedies) that we have learned from our ancestors.

On the other hand, few females mentioned that some of them visit homeopathic doctors and spiritual leaders to get some spiritual amulets because they think that they are suffering from Jin (ghost).

"We go according to our affordability, sometimes we don't go to the hospital we just deliver the baby at home (Female of the community)"

"We treat our self at home. We arrange packets and drink those at home" (Female of the community).

Dietary practices of rural women

Current dietary practices of pregnant women

Most men and women reported that as soon as the pregnancy news is heard in the family, mother-in-laws offer some specific dairy food items to pregnant women including, milk, yogurt, butter, and beverage of yogurt [lassi in local language], to prevent weakness and fatigue in women. Few women verbalized that intake of vegetables such as green chili spinach, brinjal, cauliflower, ridge gourd, tomato, potato, pumpkin, and ladyfinger is also preferred during pregnancy. Besides, women also highlighted that they try to have different food items every day, and sometimes, their menu includes protein-rich foods including fish, meat, and pulses. On the contrary, few women mentioned that because they are poor and uneducated, they eat whatever is easily available. Additionally, both men and women informed that pregnant women usually prefer to eat chili bread and do not consume fruits very often, due to the affordability issue. On the inquiring number of meals per day, few women mentioned that they don't eat at all three times; they only consume food when they are hungry.

Besides, both men and women were of opinion that pregnant women are addicted to chewable tobacco [ghutka/mawa/chura in local language] during pregnancy, which tends to decrease their appetite, leading to reduced food and nutrient intake, and consequently causing weakness and fatigue. Few men highlighted that tobacco makes up 80% of the pregnant women's diet and further explained that while they go out for the purchase of regular grocery items; their wives insist them to bring ghutka. Few women mentioned that most pregnant women usually like consuming fuller's earth [multani mud in local language], due to its taste and smell, which eventually leads to blood deficiency. One male verbalized that most women leave for farms and agriculture fields after consuming morning tea and return at lunchtime to consume chili bread. Men further highlighted that this routine could affect mother and child health outcomes.

Healthcare providers including doctors mentioned that consuming tobacco is very common among pregnant women. Doctors further emphasized that most pregnant women believe that consumption of tobacco provides energy and strength. Doctors further stated that sadly these behaviors and habits are even transferred to the born baby as well. One of the health care providers highlighted that there is gender discrimination our district and sons are given more importance as compared to daughters. Sons even ask for poison (Ghutka) to eat, parents will provide them. Parents feel proud of their sons demanding Ghutka because they think their child is growing older and demanding Gutka.

Health providers reported that women usually do not take proper nutrition. Unlike urban areas, where women eat thrice a day during, rural pregnant women usually have only two meals per day, one in the morning and one in the evening around 0700pm. One health care provider stated that even though women have easy access to vegetables in the fields, they do not prefer to eat themselves rather they sell in the market to earn money. One TBA stated that women are very much addicted to tobacco and fuller's earth, and therefore it is very difficult for them to discontinue this behavior for future pregnancies.

"Eating gutka is very common in females. Every mother is eating gutka herself, even they are feeding those habits to the baby as well who is still in their lap (Health care providers)"

"In villages children who do not have a complete number of teeth are also eating Gutka" (Health Care providers).

Recommended dietary practices to prevent anemia

Females of the communities think that juices and fruits such as apple, banana, and pomegranate are essential to alleviate anemia. In addition, women verbalized that poultry items such as chicken, fish, and eggs are also important for pregnant women to meet additional nutrient requirements. However, women voiced that they did not like eating such foods, therefore they try to avoid it during meals. Some women reported that dairy products such as milk and vegetables including spinach, eggplant, bottle gourd, and ladyfinger make a healthy pregnancy diet.

Most of the health care providers recommended that the nutrition of pregnant mothers should be proper and they should eat with other family members rather than eating leftovers at the end. Women should be told to use available dietary resources to meet their requirements such as eating dates and spinach. We cannot recommend them to use supplements such as powder milk or calcium supplements (CAC 1000), therefore we advise them to use their available sources such as cucumber and dates. It is better to eat a bowl of spinach rather than taking these supplements of iron in the form of injections. Secondly, the main thing is to focus on the education of children from beginning and children should be taught about the benefits of adequate nutrition and the harmful effects of Ghuttka. Unfortunately, we have school buildings but no one is monitoring either teacher are giving proper education or not.

> *"Out of twenty children, if five get a good education, they can bring some change"* *(Health care provider).*

> *"In winters, family members give dates and oil to cattle but don't give this to the females"(Health care provider).*

> *"1 ampule of jectofer (Iron injection) is equal to 1 bowl of Spinach and this will save your doctor fee, transportation expense and also give benefit because it's natural food(Health care provider)*

Hurdles in adopting healthy food practices

Men of the households stated that poor quality food is available in the markets and because of that women are prone to develop anemia during pregnancy. In addition, males reported that clean water is also not available for drinking purposes and therefore they have to use tap water, which is again a major cause for anemia among women of reproductive age.   One TBA highlighted that medication is not used to treat anemia among pregnant women as they do not have sufficient financial resources.

One of the health care providers highlighted that people have become greedy to earn more money and they sell all fresh things (desi eggs, pure milk) to others. If we recall our past and practices of forefathers, they used to bring the newborn child to the villages to have fresh air and fresh food. But now a day, villagers have become greedy for money and sell out all fresh things such as honey, milk, and eggs to others. They do not realize that same things can be beneficial for them as well. This money is being used to purchase unhealthy foods such as Ghutka for their family members.

> *"People come from cities, and collect all the fresh items from villagers and also give them a schedule for the next delivery'. (Health care provider)*

Knowledge and practices for Iron–Folic Acid (IFA) supplements usage

Men and women in rural communities think that small yellow tablets (Folic acid), black tablets (ferrous sulphate), syrups (syngobion), and red or brown capsules are usually advised by doctors and TBAs for anemia. Females mentioned that doctors prescribed them half white and half yellow tablets and syrup in the yellow bottle. Males further voiced that women take the prescribed medicines, as advised by doctors, as it helps in making the blood in the body. Males expressed

29

that, nowadays tablets are commonly used during pregnancy to ensure that women are having healthy pregnancy. Health care providers mentioned that we provide iron and folic acid to mothers from the stock of government hospitals and they use them if given proper guidance. One of the health care providers mentioned that I ask females to bring used wrappers back to health care providers to ensure compliance.

One of the health care providers verbalized that women consider Iron and folic acid as tiny useless tablets and sometimes they throw it without using. When we provide these tablets to women coming to us from far-flung areas, they just throw these tables. They would say that we have not come to your clinics from remote areas to get these tiny tablets and we can get these from our native towns. Therefore, health care providers and LHWs should counsel them about their importance.

> *"We have spent too much time and money to visit your clinic not to get these tiny and useless tables". (Health Care Provider)*

Reasons for compliance or non-compliance

TBAs believe that limited financial resources are the major reason for non-compliance to iron and folic acid supplements in pregnancy. Additionally, TBAs mentioned that there are only a few families who can afford charges for treatment and hospital admission.

Further, TBAs also think that there are many such cases in the village, who don't go to health facilities due to affordability issues. In case, if pregnant women suffer from heavy blood loss, then she is taken to the health facility for blood transfusion. In addition, due to lack of awareness and illiteracy, pregnant females do not take prescribed medication for 9 months and they take it very lightly. Health care providers also highlighted that people in our area do not have feelings and husbands of women also do not bother their wives and usually consider that if a woman or child dies it is the wish of God, not their fault. For example, if we advise males that your wife is anemic and you should take care of her from the beginning otherwise she will need a blood transfusion or might die. They respond by saying that its fine and we will visit your clinic for blood transfusion when required. Even if the hospital gives them any medication or support, they do not give them importance. One of the doctors mentioned that lady health workers (LHWs) provide Iron and folic acid to the women at doorsteps but they do not follow them to ensure compliance with the supplements. In addition, government officers are also not working properly and do not have enough time to counsel or follow women.

> *"Educated people of urban areas are even not smart; they buy iron during pregnancies but they don't take those medications (Health Care provider) ."*

"If 8 children of a couple got expired in the past that is not an issue for them, they will produce another one. God forbid if, during ninth pregnancy a woman dies, the husband does not worry about her and simply says this is the wish of GOD" (Health Care Provider).

Determintants of prevention and control of anemia

Lack of desirable resources, and support of health care providers
Most men reported that sometimes women need a blood transfusion during delivery, however health facilities are not equipped with necessary resources. In addition, men verbalized that medicine is also not available in hospitals and nearby stores. Further, women during the interviews reported that the hospital charges a huge amount for labs that we are unable to afford. Also, paramedical staff also demands some amount as commission in return for providing health care, which again adds burden on the family.

Health care providers highlighted that women are not being counseled properly by most of the providers. Even If they counsel, they do not counsel couples as a whole rather they focus on women only. Moreover, counseling for postnatal care is not being emphasized by the health care providers which can prevent lots of problems if taken seriously. Government institutions have also the same problems and doctors practicing their also do not counsel mothers on the number of antenatal visits, their benefits and required investigations to be done. They only perform ultrasound and send females back home without proper counseling and ultrasound is necessary but not sufficient to tell the complete story of mother and baby. If doctors properly screen and treat anemia, then women will not have any issue during delivery and during the postnatal period, females can be saved from anemia by adequate nutrition and adequate counseling.

One of the health care providers highlighted that sometimes a woman comes to the clinic to get treatment but unfortunately she takes away many other infections and health problems from the hospital due to limited facilities. For example, a woman who gets blood transfusion will end up having hepatitis B, C, and HIV-AIDS due to unscreened blood at the hospitals or clinics. In an emergency (life and death situation), one can transfuse blood to save the life of a woman but in routine transfusion without screening is a stupid behavior but this is a common practice. Recently two deaths have been reported from Civil Hospital due to blood transfusion. In addition, during C-sections, health care providers do not use separate equipment for confirmed cases of Hepatitis C or HIV, and infection is transferred very easily from one patient to another.

In addition to this, many health care providers are not able to read and interpret the investigations such as complete blood count (CBC) of the female. How they can diagnose anemia and treat it if they are unable to interpret the reports?

"When we visit hospitals for C-sections and a woman dies due to bleeding because we cannot afford blood transfusion. Mother has blood deficiency mostly after three children. A female can only get blood if her family can afford to pay the cost of blood otherwise most people who are living here cannot afford so their females die. (Males)"

"Nowadays doctors are sitting in their clinics and assess around 300 to 400 patients per day in their clinics which is fine, but at least they should guide and counsel them properly" (Health Care Provider).

Ultrasound can assess the condition of the baby, but what about the mother? (Health Care Provider)

Sometimes, we do not know whether we are using the blood of human beings or some dead animals because most of the blood banks are not registered and provide unscreened blood to women (Health Care Provider).

Absence of government initiatives to prevent anemia

Men and women perceive that there is poor government support for health-related matters. Public hospitals do not provide adequate facilities to families who are unable to afford proper treatment and medicine charges. Women also stated that if they report to the emergency, they are being with huge amount, which they are unable to pay on discharge. Men suggested that government should provide free medicine and ban Gukta to improve the health conditions of the district. Men also highlighted that government is mostly making efforts for urban areas, and therefore rural population remains poor and unhealthy. Lastly, health care providers highlighted that although government has initiated few trainings on antenatal checkups but so far government has not worked on anemia specific programs. They further mentioned that government should arrange counselling sessions, gather male villagers and sensitize them about adequate dies and family planning. However, government has organized many trainings to handle obstetrical complications, antenatal care but it has not done anything for anemia. Unfortunately, anemia has not been given much importance by government or Non-government organizations and we should study anemia in depth and doctors should be given relevant trainings to address this major issue.

One of the health care providers mentioned that government should not only arrange trainings for health care providers but also for women in the villages. Government need to prioritize the issues and take step by step approach to resolve those issues. Government and nongovernment organizations should organize role plays, sessions and seminars for beneficiaries such as villagers rather than only training health care providers.

"They should ban using ghutkas and other things that cause blood deficiency if people will save money than they can utilize in buying good things. (Female of the community)"

"They should provide free medicines and built nearby hospitals" (Female of the community)

"Government only works in cities, not in villages. The government has banned mawa, but what is happening in villages? (Male of the community)"

Fragile social networks

Most females verbalized that we do not have social support from our leaders. Our leaders (Wadera) do not look into the problems faced by us and they do not help us. We manage all things by ourselves. For instance, if someone is suffering from any disease at our home, we arrange transport and take them to the hospital ourselves. Our leaders are not concerned about us they only rule us and show their power. In addition, leaders are mostly busy with their work and they are leaders by name only. They don't provide us anything; they just come for a vote at the time of the election. During rainy days, they don't care for us and don't provide us electricity as well. When we need any help, leaders just disappeared and there is no one to listen to our complaints. Only you are asking us about our health and interviewing us otherwise this, no one else is working on health problems.

> *"Community leaders do not bother even if a woman dies in the village. They wait for another day to come and forget about the dead woman". (Female of the community)*

Financial barriers

On inquiring about financial barriers, most men stated that they are poor and therefore they are unable to provide proper food to the family. Men suggested that the government should provide employment opportunities so that they can earn and improve their financial conditions. Health providers reported that due to poverty in the district, women also have to work in the fields for long hours and therefore their food and health gets compromised.

Females also mentioned that we are aware of the fact that we should eat fresh milk and butter but we cannot afford it. They also highlighted that health care providers should not charge their fees as we are poor. They should rather give us benefits and provide us medicines free of cost. If the mother cannot afford treatment and does not visit doctors then she dies. Females also mentioned that leaders in their communities should provide them opportunities for earning such as developing their skills to earn for their families.

One of the females mentioned that I have been sick for the last six months, I have lots of tensions and we have just one earning person in our family. I have blood deficiency too and everyone advises me to eat fruits and vegetables to have some energy. I went to the doctor but her treatment was very expensive and she advised me to administer a drip that costs around 2000 RS and I cannot afford that expensive treatment. One of the health care providers mentioned that usually, patients coming to them are too poor to afford to buy fruits or iron-rich foods for them. TBAs verbalized that poor people are not able to eat proper food as they cannot afford to purchase food. One of the TBAs mentioned that when we take an anemic woman to the facility or clinic, doctor advice for blood transfusion. Everyone cannot afford blood transfusion as some are poor and some are rich.

> *"Rich families can afford blood transfusion to address the issue of blood deficiency among women but poor people cannot afford" (Health Care provider).*

"If health care providers or government provide us benefits then we will do whatever they will advise". (Female)

"Doctors refers us to the hospitals and we take loan from others in order to get treatment" (Female).

Interval between subsequent pregnancies

On inquiring about frequent pregnancies and family planning, mixed responses were reported by both males and females. Females reported that people should avoid contraceptives especially injections as this causes several problems such as bleeding, weight gain, dizziness, etc. Few mothers reported that getting pregnant every year is normal and that does not cause anemia. Males of the community reported that they do not have an idea about family planning. However, few males and females reported that a proper gap and spacing between pregnancies is good for mother and child health.

In addition, doctors also reported people to have several myths about family planning. If we offer post-partum family planning to mothers during labor, they think we are doing a big sin and do not give us consent for family planning. One of the health care providers mentioned that she tried to counsel a female for family planning delivering her 18th child. The woman got irritated and said that I do not want to discuss this or talk about family planning as it will result in the death of my child.

Modern and new techniques cannot work unless we create awareness among women and addresses their myths and misconceptions about family planning methods. Females need to be counseled about family planning and we might face difficulty to counsel them at the beginning but we need to start. For example, if two clients are counseled for family planning, they will bring another two clients and the circle will keep on expanding. Secondly, due to our culture, it might not be suitable to counsel women for family planning in front of their husbands. One of the TBAs also verbalized that family planning is not good for women's health. A TBA reported that if a female will ask for family planning her husband will not allow her. Most of the health care providers verbalized that women should practice family planning. If females cannot afford food, shelter, education, and clothes to wear then they should use family planning methods. In fact, women must go for ligation when their family is complete or male should go for a vasectomy.

"The woman who is getting pregnant she is better than that woman who is doing family planning (Female of the community)"

"As the first child start walking woman try for another baby (Female of the community)."

"For GOD sake, I have not given birth to my child and you are asking me to do this sin of using Family Planning method" (Health Care provider).

"GOD will be unhappy if you discuss family planning with me and God's unhappiness will result death of my child" (Health Care provider).

Chapter 4: Addressing anemia in rural Pakistan: Transforming community environment

Brief overview of anemia

Research has indicated that women of reproductive age experience a high burden of anemia in developing countries including Pakistan. Consumption of smokeless tobacco (gutka) and an inadequate diet are two important risk factors for anemia among women of reproductive age in rural Pakistan. Anemia increases the risk of maternal and perinatal adverse outcomes such as stillbirths, preterm births, low birth weight, and maternal and neonatal deaths. Therefore, community midwives and higher authorities in health, nutrition, and food and agriculture departments should work together to address the burden of anemia among women of reproductive age in Pakistan.

Gutka Usage and Inadequate Diet as Important Risk Factors of Anemia

Gutka is a type of smokeless chewable tobacco made up of areca nut, slaked lime, catechu, tobacco, flavoring agents, and sweeteners (Varghese, Swaminathan, Kurpad, & Thomas, 2019). Tobacco found in gutka decreases iron absorption and thus decreases iron stores thereby causing anemia (Mistry et al., 2018; Subramoney & Gupta, 2008). Moreover, tobacco suppresses appetite, reducing the intake of food and important micronutrients by WRA thereby increasing their susceptibility to anemia (Miyata, Meguid, Fetissov, Torelli, & Kim, 1999).

Consumption of an unhealthy diet is another important risk factor of anemia due to inadequate resources, and food insecurity in rural Pakistan (Habib et al., 2018; Ndegwa, 2019). I have personally seen that rural men in Pakistan work on the farms to grow vegetables and fruits rich in iron, and many also have livestock. Unfortunately, these men do not allow WRA to eat these vegetables, fruits, and dairy products they are rather sold in the city to earn money.

Anemia affects WRA, their children, and families (Kumar, Asha, Murthy, Sujatha, & Manjunath, 2013; Rahmati, Delpishe, Azami, Ahmadi, & Sayehmiri, 2017). In addition, gutka usage is common in poor communities and buying gutka from the market further drags WRA down into poverty (Sinha et al., 2013). This prevents women to purchase healthy food for themselves thus further deteriorating their health and thereby increasing their chances of anemia. Considering the adverse effects of anemia due to gutka and inadequate diet, there is a need for transformation by addressing these two risk factors. This will not only improve the health of WRA but also their children in rural Pakistan.

Recommendations to Reduce Gutka and Improve Adequate diet

Two strategies will help WRA to change their behavior by reducing gutka consumption and eat a healthy diet in a sustainable way. The first strategy is to train CMWs and bridge them between communities and higher authorities in the health care system. Studies revealed that CMWs being highly respected members of the community have played a crucial role in reaching hard-to-access areas, the poor, and marginalized communities (Abimbola, Okoli, Olubajo, Abdullahi, & Pate, 2012; Wangmo et al., 2016). Another strategy is to help WRA to grow kitchen gardens and also aid them to get microloans to purchase livestock. Evidence suggests that kitchen gardens can improve the nutritional security in households in a sustainable manner (Arya, Prakash, Joshi, Tripathi, & Singh, 2018; Mohsin, Anwar, Jamal, Ajmal, & Breuste, 2017). These two proposed strategies will be piloted in one district followed by scaling up these strategies across all rural areas of Pakistan.

Proposed Plan for Recommended Transformation

To operationalize the proposed strategies, collaboration with the national program on Maternal, Newborn and Child Health (MNCH) of Pakistan is essential. One of the main objectives of the MNCH program is to train and deploy CMWs to serve WRA in remote areas (Mumtaz, Levay, & Bhatti, 2015). These CMWs are 16 to 35-year-old married females, have a minimum of ten years' education, and have experience of working in the communities (Ali et al., 2015). After recruiting CMWs, the MNCH program provides them training for 18 months to develop their skills for providing health care services in rural areas. The Pakistan nursing council is the overall nursing body of CMWs (Ali et al., 2015). To date, 8000 CMWs have been trained and deployed in different rural areas of Pakistan (Mumtaz, Levay, & Bhatti, 2015).

These proposed strategies need to be integrated into the MCNH program so that the program can bear the cost of these strategies and also take responsibility for implementing these in a sustainable manner. The first step would be to list all CMWs, who have completed their basic 18 months training and have started working in different rural areas of Pakistan. This will be followed by organizing an advanced two weeks training workshop in collaboration with the MNCH program to train CMWs on five main themes to enable them working effectively in communities. These themes include understanding community dynamics, communication, and interpersonal skills, bridging between the community and higher authorities, decision making, and advocacy. The training will consist of in-class sessions and practical exercises by showing videos to CMWs on different themes, engaging them in role-playing, and discussing case studies.

After training, CMWs will schedule to visit WRA at their homes on a monthly basis. CMWs will make support groups of WRA in each village. These support groups will meet with CMWs once a month but they will continue to meet each other on a weekly basis. During meetings, CMWs will understand the reasons for using gutka by WRA and will explain to them the adverse effects of gutka. Moreover, CMWs will give health education messages to WRA, show videos in the local language on the adverse effects of gutka and will provide them alternatives to gutka such as using chew gums to slowly reduce consumption of gutka. Behavior change is a constant and gradual process that needs consistent reminders and motivation (Siddiqi et al., 2016). Therefore, CMWs will ask support groups to run these community meetings, when CMWs are not around.

Male members are the main purchasers of gutka from the market and they also bring gutka for their wives. Therefore, CMWs will also meet with male members of the villages to educate them about the importance of the health of WRA. They will encourage men to stop purchasing gutka and promote investing the same money to grow kitchen gardens.

The second strategy is to help women develop kitchen gardens by making CMWs as bridges between communities and officials of health, nutrition, finance and food, and agriculture departments. CMWs will meet with officials of these departments to make them aware of the burden of anemia and gutka usage by WRA, advocate for the health of women by liaising with three departments and will plan to grow kitchen gardens for women.

While meeting with officials of different departments, CMWs will motivate them to release the budget for developing kitchen gardens and purchasing livestock. CMWs will explain to these departments about the importance of growing kitchen gardens as sustainable, cost-effective, and self-sufficient strategies. This will prevent women from becoming dependent upon outside short term nutritional support from different donors in the form of nutritional sachets or supplements. CMWs will work closely with nutrition and agriculture departments to design strategies to help WRA to grow kitchen gardens in their homes.

In addition, women will also need livestock to consume dairy products along with vegetables and fruits. This will require investing some money initially and CMWs will request the finance department to give microloans to these women. These microloans will help women to purchase material for kitchen gardens and livestock for dairy products. In addition, CMWs will motivate male members to grow iron-rich foods on their farms, which should not only be sold in the cities but also allow WRA to use those foods in their diets.

Conclusion

Community midwives can become a bridge between communities and higher authorities to raise voice for anemic WRA of rural Pakistan. CMWs will closely work with women in communities and also liaison with health, nutrition, and food and agriculture departments to address the burden of anemia through addressing problems of gutka, and an inadequate diet. Thus, CMWs will help women to change their behavior to stop using gutka and consume a healthy diet from their own kitchen gardens, which can be sustainable and cost-effective strategies to reduce the burden of anemia among WRA of rural Pakistan.

References

Abimbola, S., Okoli, U., Olubajo, O., Abdullahi, M. J., & Pate, M. A. (2012). The midwives service scheme in Nigeria. *PLoS Medicine, 9*(5), e1001211.

Ali, S. A., Lakhani, A., Jan, R., Shahid, S., Baig, M., & Adnan, F. (2015). Enhancement of knowledge and skills of community midwives in Sindh, Pakistan. *Journal of Asian Midwives (JAM)*, *2*(2), 36-56.

Arora, M., Tewari, A., Tripathy, V., Nazar, G. P., Juneja, N. S., Ramakrishnan, L., & Reddy, K. S. (2010). Community-based model for preventing tobacco use among disadvantaged adolescents in urban slums of India. *Health Promotion International*, *25*(2), 143-152.

Arya, S., Prakash, S., Joshi, S., Tripathi, K. M., & Singh, V. (2018). Household food security through kitchen gardening in Rural Areas of Western Uttar Pradesh, India. *International Journal Current Microbiology Applied Sciences*, *7*(2), 468-474.

Beckert, R. H., Baer, R. J., Anderson, J. G., Jelliffe-Pawlowski, L. L., & Rogers, E. E. (2019). Maternal anemia and pregnancy outcomes: A population-based study. *Journal of Perinatology*, *39*, 911-919. doi:10.1038/s41372-019-0375-0

Bittencourt, L., & Scarinci, I. C. (2014). Is there a role for community midwives in tobacco cessation programs? Perceptions of administrators and health care professionals. *Nicotine & Tobacco Research*, *16*(5), 626-631.

Bloch, M., Althabe, F., Onyamboko, M., Kaseba-Sata, C., Castilla, E. E., Freire, S., ... & Goco, N. (2008). Tobacco use and secondhand smoke exposure during pregnancy: An investigative survey of women in 9 developing nations. *American Journal of Public Health*, *98*(10), 1833-1840.

Cappellini, M. D., & Motta, I. (2015). Anemia in clinical practice-definition and classification: Does hemoglobin change with aging? *Seminars Hematology*, *52*(4)261-269. doi:10.1053/j.seminhematol.2015.07.006.

Habib, M. A., Raynes-Greenow, C., Soofi, S. B., Ali, N., Nausheen, S., Ahmed, I., . . . Black, K. I. (2018). Prevalence and determinants of iron deficiency anemia among non-pregnant women of reproductive age in Pakistan. *Asia Pacific Journal of Clinical Nutrition*, *27*(1), 195. doi: 10.6133/apjcn.042017.14.

Javed, F., Chotai, M., Mehmood, A., & Almas, K. (2010). Oral mucosal disorders associated with habitual gutka usage: A review. *Oral Surgery, Oral Medicine, Oral Pathology, Oral Radiology, and Endodontology*, *109*(6), 857-864.

Kumar, K. J., Asha, N., Murthy, D. S., Sujatha, M. S., & Manjunath, V. G. (2013). Maternal anemia in various trimesters and its effect on newborn weight and maturity: An observational study. *International Journal of Preventive Medicine*, *4*(2), 193.

Lander, R. L., Hambidge, K. M., Westcott, J. E., Tejeda, G., Diba, T. S., Mastiholi, S. C., ... & Lokangaka, A. (2019). Pregnant women in four low-middle income countries have a high prevalence of inadequate dietary intakes that are improved by dietary diversity. *Nutrients, 11*(7), 1560.

Mason, J., Martorell, R., Saldanha, L., & Shrimpton, R. (2013). Reduction of anaemia. *The Lancet Global Health, 1*(1), e4-e6.

Mistry, R., Jones, A. D., Pednekar, M. S., Dhumal, G., Dasika, A., Kulkarni, U., . . . Gupta, P. C. (2018). Antenatal tobacco use and iron deficiency anemia: integrating tobacco control into antenatal care in urban India. *Reproductive Health, 15*(1), 72.

Miyata, G., Meguid, M. M., Fetissov, S. O., Torelli, G. F., & Kim, H.-J. (1999). Nicotine's effect on hypothalamic neurotransmitters and appetite regulation. *Surgery, 126*(2), 255-263.

Mohsin, M., Anwar, M. M., Jamal, F., Ajmal, F., & Breuste, J. (2017). Assessing the role and effectiveness of kitchen gardening toward food security in Punjab, Pakistan: A case of district Bahawalpur. *International Journal of Urban Sustainable Development, 9*(1), 64-78.

Mumtaz, Z., Levay, A. V., & Bhatti, A. (2015). Successful community midwives in Pakistan: An asset-based approach. *PloS one, 10*(9), e0135302.

Ndegwa, S. K. (2019). Anemia and its associated factors among pregnant women attending antenatal clinic at Mbagathi County Hospital, Nairobi County, Kenya. *African Journal of Health Sciences, 32*(1), 59-73.

Parks, S., Hoffman, M. K., Goudar, S. S., Patel, A., Saleem, S., Ali, S. A., . . . Wallace, D.

(2019). Maternal anemia and maternal, fetal, and neonatal outcomes in a prospective cohort study in India and Pakistan. *An International Journal of Obstetrics & Gynaecology. 126*(6), 737-743. doi: 10.1111/1471.

Rahmati, S., Delpishe, A., Azami, M., Ahmadi, M. R. H., & Sayehmiri, K. (2017). Maternal Anemia during pregnancy and infant low birth weight: A systematic review and Meta-analysis. *International Journal of Reproductive BioMedicine, 15*(3), 125.

Rukuni, R., Bhattacharya, S., Murphy, M. F., Roberts, D., Stanworth, S. J., & Knight, M. (2016). Maternal and neonatal outcomes of antenatal anemia in a Scottish population: A retrospective cohort study. *Acta Obstetrics Gynecology Scandinavian, 95*(5), 555-564. doi:10.1111/aogs.12862.

Siddiqi, K., Dogar, O., Rashid, R., Jackson, C., Kellar, I., O'Neill, N., . . . Thomson, H. (2016). Behaviour change intervention for smokeless tobacco cessation: its development, feasibility and fidelity testing in Pakistan and in the UK. *BMC public health, 16*(1), 501.

Sinha, D. N., Gupta, P. C., Kumar, A., Bhartiya, D., Agarwal, N., Sharma, S., ... & Mehrotra, R. (2017). The poorest of the poor suffer the greatest burden from smokeless tobacco use: A study from 140 countries. *Nicotine and Tobacco Research, 20*(12), 1529-1532.

Stevens, G. A., Finucane, M. M., De-Regil, L. M., Paciorek, C. J., Flaxman, S. R., Branca, F., ... & Nutrition Impact Model Study Group. (2013). Global, regional, and national trends in hemoglobin concentration and prevalence of total and severe anemia in children and pregnant and non-pregnant women for 1995–2011: A systematic analysis of population-representative data. *The Lancet Global Health, 1*(1), e16-e25.

Subramoney, S., & Gupta, P. C. (2008). Anemia in pregnant women who use smokeless tobacco. *Nicotine & tobacco research, 10*(5), 917-920.

Tunkyi, K., & Moodley, J. (2018). Anemia and pregnancy outcomes: A longitudinal study. *The Journal of Maternal-Fetal & Neonatal Medicine, 31*(19), 2594-2598. doi:10.1080/14767058.2017.1349746.

United Nations International Children's Emergency Fund. (2019, June). National nutrition survey 2018-key findings report. Retrieved from https://www.unicef.org/pakistan/reports/national-nutrition-survey-2018-key-findings-.

Varghese, J. S., Swaminathan, S., Kurpad, A. V., & Thomas, T. (2019). Demand and supply factors of iron-folic acid supplementation and its association with anaemia in North Indian pregnant women. *PloS one, 14*(1), e0210634.

Wangmo, S., Suphanchaimat, R., Htun, W. M. M., Aung, T. T., Khitdee, C., Patcharanarumol, W., . . . Tangcharoensathien, V. (2016). Auxiliary midwives in hard to reach rural areas of Myanmar: filling MCH gaps. *BMC public health, 16*(1), 914.

Youssry, M. A., Radwan, A. M., Gebreel, M. A., & Patel, T. A. (2018). Prevalence of maternal anemia in pregnancy: The effect of maternal hemoglobin level on pregnancy and neonatal outcome. *Open Journal of Obstetrics and Gynecology, 8*(07), 676.

1.   Kamruzzaman M, Rabbani MG, Saw A, Sayem MA, Hossain MG. Differentials in the prevalence of anemia among non-pregnant, ever-married women in Bangladesh: multilevel logistic regression analysis of data from the 2011 Bangladesh Demographic and Health Survey. BMC women's health. 2015;15(1):54.

2.   Chowdhury HA, Ahmed KR, Jebunessa F, Akter J, Hossain S, Shahjahan M. Factors associated with maternal anaemia among pregnant women in Dhaka city. BMC women's health. 2015;15(1):77.

3.   Lover AA, Hartman M, Chia KS, Heymann DL. Demographic and spatial predictors of anemia in women of reproductive age in Timor-Leste: implications for health program prioritization. PLoS One. 2014;9(3):e91252.

4.   Ullah I, Zahid M, Khan MI, Shah M. Prevalence of anemia in pregnant women in district Karak, Khyber Pakhtunkhwa, Pakistan. International Journal of Biosciences. 2013;3:77-83.

5.   Page CM, Patel A, Hibberd PL. Does smoke from biomass fuel contribute to anemia in pregnant women in Nagpur, India? A cross-sectional study. PloS one. 2015;10(5):e0127890.

6.   McClure EM, Meshnick SR, Mungai P, Malhotra I, King CL, Goldenberg RL, et al. The association of parasitic infections in pregnancy and maternal and fetal anemia: a cohort study in coastal Kenya. PLoS neglected tropical diseases. 2014;8(2):e2724.

7.   Addis Alene K, Mohamed Dohe A. Prevalence of anemia and associated factors among pregnant women in an urban area of Eastern Ethiopia. Anemia. 2014;2014.

8.   Habib MA, Raynes-Greenow C, Soofi SB, Ali N, Nausheen S, Ahmed I, et al. Prevalence and determinants of iron deficiency anemia among non-pregnant women of reproductive age in Pakistan. Asia Pacific journal of clinical nutrition. 2018;27(1):195.

9.   Getachew M, Yewhalaw D, Tafess K, Getachew Y, Zeynudin A. Anaemia and associated risk factors among pregnant women in Gilgel Gibe dam area, Southwest Ethiopia. Parasites & vectors. 2012;5(1):296.

10.   Baig-Ansari N, Badruddin SH, Karmaliani R, Harris H, Jehan I, Pasha O, et al. Anemia prevalence and risk factors in pregnant women in an urban area of Pakistan. Food and nutrition bulletin. 2008;29(2):132-9.

11.   Kedir H, Berhane Y, Worku A. Khat chewing and restrictive dietary behaviors are associated with anemia among pregnant women in high prevalence rural communities in eastern Ethiopia. PLoS One. 2013;8(11):e78601.

12.   Ononge S, Campbell O, Mirembe F. Haemoglobin status and predictors of anaemia among pregnant women in Mpigi, Uganda. BMC research notes. 2014;7(1):712.

13.   Haidar J. Prevalence of anaemia, deficiencies of iron and folic acid and their determinants in Ethiopian women. Journal of health, population, and nutrition. 2010;28(4):359.

Publisher: Eliva Press SRL

Email: info@elivapress.com